AVITAL SILVERBERG

SKINNY MINDSET

Copyright © 2023 by Avital Silverberg

All rights reserved. No part of this publication may be reproduced, stored or transmitted in any form or by any means, electronic, mechanical, photocopying, recording, scanning, or otherwise without written permission from the publisher. It is illegal to copy this book, post it to a website, or distribute it by any other means without permission.

First edition

Preface

Have you ever wondered why some people seem to have an effortless ability to maintain a healthy weight, no matter what they eat or how much they exercise? So did I. I know what it's like to feel defeated and hopeless in the battle against weight, diet, and exercise.

For years, I struggled with weight loss and dieting. I tried every diet and exercise regime under the sun, but nothing seemed to work for me. In fact, it seemed like the more I tried, the worse it got. As I got older, my weight became more of an issue, and it started affecting my confidence and self-esteem. It wasn't until I developed bulimia and binge eating disorder that I realized something had to change.

For three years, I struggled with these disorders, trying to find a way out. It wasn't a simple solution that worked for me. Instead, it was a combination of approaches that finally helped me start on the road to recovery. The biggest change came when I was able to convince myself that I was capable and worthy, regardless of my weight.

I had to work on removing the values I had associated with food and my body image. Instead, I focused on inner growth and building a strong sense of self-worth. Once I stopped worrying so much about my weight, diet, and exercise, I started to see changes. I started to lose weight, eat healthier, and enjoy exercise for the first time in my life.

That's why I created this workbook. I wanted to put together all the practical tools that helped me overcome my problems with eating and weight loss. I wanted to make it easy for people to take action immediately, and reinforce some of the truths and mind tricks that helped me learn to love myself.

The term "Skinny Mindset" has nothing to do with being thin or adhering to societal norms. Instead, it's about a healthy relationship with food, our body, and our mind. It's about listening to our bodies' hunger and fullness signals and making food choices that are nourishing and satisfying. It's about viewing exercise as a fun and enjoyable way to take care of our bodies, rather than a punishment for not being thin enough. It's about challenging the negative self-talk that has been holding us back and developing a more positive and compassionate mindset.

This book is designed to introduce you to the Skinny Mindset principles, but it's also designed to reinforce them and turn them into a habit. You'll be working together with me to change your mindset and develop a healthier relationship with your body, your food, and your life.

I'll share with you the practical tools and exercises that helped me overcome my problems with eating and weight loss. We'll work together to change the way you think about food and your body, so you can achieve lasting results. We'll develop a positive self-image and a sense of self-worth and self-confidence that will help you in all areas of your life.

I know how difficult it can be to struggle with weight and body image issues, and I know how much it can affect your life. But I also know that there is a way out, and it's through the Skinny Mindset. Let's start this transformation together!

Contents

Introduction	1
Overview of the Skinny Mindset	3
Why Changing Your Mindset is Key to Losing Weight	6
The Mind-Body Weight Loss Worksheet	8
Developing a Positive Mindset	25
Letting Go of Dieting and Embracing Intuitive Eating	66
Cultivating Gratitude and Positive Body Image	77
Overcoming Emotional Eating and Cravings	83
The Importance of Mindful Eating	87
How to Practice Mindful Eating and Movement	90
Developing a Growth Mindset	94
Staying Committed to the Skinny Mindset with a	98
Growth... Recap of the Skinny Mindset Principles	128
Final Thoughts and Encouragement	131

Introduction

Hello and Welcome!

"Skinny Mindset: A Practical Guide and Worksheet to Sustainable and Lifelong Weight Loss" is a comprehensive guide designed to help you achieve your weight loss goals in a sustainable and lifelong manner. This book is more than just a traditional weight loss guide, it serves as a journal and workbook, filled with practical tasks and exercises that will help you immediately apply the knowledge and research contained within its pages.

In this book, you will discover a new way of thinking about weight loss that goes beyond the traditional approach of counting calories and exercise. Instead, "Skinny Mindset" focuses on the mental and emotional aspects of weight loss, exploring the reasons why you may have struggled with weight loss in the past and providing you with the tools to overcome these obstacles and achieve lasting success.

Whether you are a seasoned dieter or just starting your weight loss journey, this book is for you. It is written in a clear and concise manner, making it easy to understand and follow. The exercises and worksheets contained within its pages are designed to help you develop a deeper understanding of your thoughts, feelings, and habits surrounding food and exercise, and to provide you with the tools you need to make lasting changes.

"Skinny Mindset" covers a wide range of topics, including the science of weight loss, the importance of mindfulness and self-awareness, and the role of positive self-talk and visualization in achieving your goals. You will also learn how to set realistic goals, how to develop a healthy relationship with food, and how to cultivate a supportive network of friends and family who will encourage and motivate you along the way.

So if you are ready to take control of your weight and achieve the body you've always wanted, grab a copy of "Skinny Mindset: A Practical Guide and Worksheet to Sustainable and Lifelong Weight Loss" and start your journey to a healthier, happier, and more confident you today!

Overview of the Skinny Mindset

The Skinny Mindset is a weight loss program that is built on the principle that the key to successful weight loss lies in the power of the mind. It is a revolutionary approach that recognizes the importance of both the mind and the body in the weight loss process, and provides a holistic solution to help you achieve your weight loss goals.

The power of the Skinny Mindset lies in its ability to help you shift your perspective on weight loss and your relationship with food and your body. This mindset shift is critical because it is often our negative thoughts and beliefs about ourselves, our bodies, and food that hold us back from achieving our weight loss goals. By changing our thoughts and beliefs, we can change our behavior and achieve the results we desire.

The Skinny Mindset provides a framework for addressing the mental and emotional aspects of weight loss, which are often ignored in traditional weight loss programs. It helps you identify the roadblocks that have been holding you back and provides you with tools and techniques to overcome them. For example, if you struggle with emotional eating, the Skinny Mindset will provide you with strategies to help you manage your emotions without relying on food.

One of the key principles of the Skinny Mindset is the importance of self-talk and affirmations. Our self-talk is the internal dialogue that we have with ourselves, and it can have a powerful impact on our weight loss efforts. If we have negative thoughts about ourselves, our bodies, and food, it can lead to feelings of self-doubt and low self-esteem, which can make it difficult to stick to a healthy eating plan. The Skinny Mindset teaches you how to replace negative self-talk with positive affirmations that will help you feel confident and empowered in your weight loss journey.

Another powerful aspect of the Skinny Mindset is its emphasis on mindful eating and movement. Mindful eating involves paying at-tention to the sensations of hunger and fullness, and eating without distractions. By practicing mindful eating, you will become more in tune with your body's natural signals, which will help you make healthier food choices and avoid overeating. The Skinny Mindset also emphasizes the importance of movement and physical activity, and provides strategies to help you incorporate exercise into your daily routine in a way that is enjoyable and sustainable.

In conclusion, the power of the Skinny Mindset lies in its ability to help you shift your perspective on weight loss and create a positive and empowering mindset that will support you in achieving your goals. By addressing the mental and emotional aspects of weight loss, the Skinny Mindset provides a comprehensive solution for lasting success. So, if you're ready to take control of your weight and your life, embrace the power of the Skinny Mindset and start your journey to a happier, healthier you.

Workbook format will help you create a personalized plan for weight loss success. And also reflect and track your progress while you are learning how to identify and overcome the mental and emotional obstacles and develop a new and empowering mindset that will support you in your weight loss journey.

With "Skinny Mindset," you will learn how to:

- Overcome emotional eating and develop a healthy relationship with food
- Identify and challenge negative thoughts and beliefs about yourself and your body
- Create a personalized and sustainable weight loss plan
- Incorporate healthy habits into your daily routine
- Build self-confidence and a positive body image

This book is not just a guide, but a complete and interactive experience. The workbook provides space for you to reflect on your thoughts, track your progress, and celebrate your accomplishments.

Why Changing Your Mindset is Key to Losing Weight

Weight loss is a complex issue that requires a multi-faceted approach to be successful. While it is well known that diet and exercise play a crucial role in weight loss, many people fail to recognize the critical role that mindset plays in the process. In fact, changing your mindset is key to losing weight and achieving long-term success.

The problem with traditional diets and weight loss programs is that they focus solely on the physical aspect of weight loss, ignoring the mental and emotional components. They often prescribe strict eating plans and exercise regimens that are difficult to stick to, leaving people feeling deprived, frustrated, and discouraged. These diets may produce short-term results, but they are often unsustainable, and people end up gaining back the weight they have lost.

This guide, on the other hand, recognizes the importance of both the mind and the body in the weight loss process and provides a holistic approach that addresses both. By changing your mindset, you will develop a positive relationship with food and your body that will support you in making healthy choices, sticking to your weight loss plan, and achieving your goals.

One of the key reasons why changing your mindset is key to losing weight is because our thoughts, beliefs, and attitudes about ourselves, our bodies, and food have a powerful impact on our behavior. Negative thoughts and beliefs can lead to feelings of self-doubt and low self-esteem, making it difficult to stick to a healthy eating plan and exercise regimen. By changing these negative thoughts and beliefs to positive ones, you can create a supportive and empowering environment that will help you stay motivated and on track.

Another reason why changing your mindset is key to losing weight is because it helps you overcome the mental and emotional roadblocks that have been holding you back. For example, if you struggle with emotional eating, then you can apply strategies that will help you manage your emotions without relying on food. By addressing the root causes of your weight loss struggles, you will be able to overcome them and achieve lasting success.

Changing your mindset is key to losing weight because it helps you cultivate a growth mindset. A growth mindset is a belief that you have the ability to grow and change, and that with effort and determination, you can achieve your goals. By embracing a growth mindset, you will be more resilient in the face of setbacks, and more likely to persevere and reach your weight loss goals.

The Mind-Body Weight Loss Worksheet

Your mindset is the collection of beliefs, attitudes, and assumptions you have about yourself and the world. This includes how you view yourself, your ability to make changes, and how you respond to challenges. Your mindset has a powerful effect on your behavior and ability to reach your goals. It can help you stay motivated, break old habits, and create new ones. It can also be a barrier that keeps you from making progress.

Acknowledge your current mindset: Before you can change your mindset, you have to acknowledge it. Identify your current beliefs, attitudes, and assumptions about yourself and the world.

Answer these questions on the following pages:

-What are your current beliefs and attitudes about weight loss?
-What are your assumptions about the process of losing weight?
-How do you see yourself in relation to your body and weight?

-How have past experiences with weight loss shaped your current mindset?
-What fears or insecurities do you have about the process of losing weight?
-How do you think your friends, family, and society influence your beliefs and attitudes towards weight loss?
-How would you describe your current level of self-esteem and body confidence?

Take some time to reflect on your life experiences. Make a list of the events, people, and places that have had the most influence on you. Ask yourself questions like "What has been my experience with this person/place/event?" or "What did I learn from this experience?"

1. How has my relationship with food and exercise changed over the years?
2. What are the triggers that lead me to overeat or make unhealthy food choices?
3. What have been my past experiences with weight loss and why were they successful or unsuccessful?
4. How have my emotions and stress levels affected my weight loss journey?
5. What are my biggest motivators and challenges in achieving my weight loss goals?
6. How do I envision my future self?

Make a list of your core values. What do you think is most important in life? What principles do you live by?

1. What is your main motivation for losing weight?
2. What are your goals for your weight loss journey?
3. How do your core values and principles impact your weight loss journey?
4. How do you plan to balance your weight loss goals with your other priorities in life?
5. What habits or behaviors do you need to change in order to reach your weight loss goals?
6. What support system do you have in place to help you stay on track with your weight loss journey?
7. How do you plan to stay accountable and maintain motivation throughout your journey?

Identify your assumptions and beliefs. Try to be as objective as possible. Ask yourself questions like "What do I assume to be true?" or "What do I believe to be true?"
1. What assumptions do I have about weight loss?
2. What are my beliefs about my own ability to lose weight?
3. Do I believe that weight loss is solely about diet and exercise?
4. Do I believe that weight loss is easy or difficult?
5. What do I believe are the causes of weight gain?
6. Do I believe that weight loss is a personal choice or is influenced by external factors?

Do you agree or disagree with following statements?

1. I believe in the power of healthy eating habits, exercise, and self-discipline

2. I believe in the power of hard work, dedication, and resilience.

3. I believe that I have the power to make positive changes in my lifestyle to achieve my goals.

4. I believe that I have the power to take risks, to learn from my mistakes, and grow.

5. I believe that I can achieve my goals if I have the right attitude and mindset.

6. I believe that I can achieve their goals if I have a clear vision and strategy.

Once you've identified your current mindset, it's time to reframe your thoughts. Look for ways to reframe negative thoughts into more positive ones. Read the examples and provide your ones below:

1. Rather than focusing on what you cannot do, focus on what you CAN do: For example, instead of focusing on the fact that you can't run a marathon, focus on the fact that you can walk for 30 minutes a day and gradually increase your exercise level.

2. Replace rigid "all-or-nothing" thinking with more flexible thinking: For example, instead of thinking that you have to complete an entire project in one day, recognize that you can work on it a little bit each day and still make progress.

3. Replace critical and judgmental self-talk with more compassionate and understanding self-talk: For example, instead of criticizing yourself for not being good at a certain task, be understanding and acknowledge that everyone has strengths and weaknesses, and that it's okay to not be good at everything.

4. Replace exaggeration ("This is the worst thing ever!") with more realistic language: For example, instead of saying "This is the worst day ever," say "Today has been a bit challenging, but I know it will get better."

5. Replace "should" and "must" statements with more forgiving "could" and "might" statements: For example, instead of saying "I should have done better," say "I could have done better, but I'm still learning and I'll do better next time."

6. Replace negative labels ("I'm a failure") with more affirming statements: For example, instead of saying "I'm a failure," say "I may have failed this time, but I am capable of success and I will keep trying."

7. Acknowledge the positives and celebrate your successes, no matter how small: For example, instead of focusing only on your failures, take the time to acknowledge and celebrate small successes, such as completing this task.

Practice self-compassion. It's important to be kind to yourself. Don't be too hard on yourself if you make mistakes or don't reach your goals. Instead, practice self-compassion and be gentle with yourself. Write your reflections on the following tasks in the space provided:

1. Task: Speak kindly to yourself.

- Write a list of 10 positive affirmations and read them to yourself every morning and evening.
- Replace negative self-talk with positive self-talk whenever it arises.
- Write down 3 things that you like about yourself every day.

2. Task: Show yourself understanding and forgiveness.

- Write a letter to yourself, forgiving yourself for any past mistakes or failures.
- Practice self-compassion by recognizing and acknowledging when you are being too hard on yourself.
- Reframe negative self-talk to be more understanding and forgiving towards yourself.

3. Task: Make time for self-care.

- Schedule a set time each week for self-care activities, such as a relaxing bath, yoga, or a massage.
- Make a list of activities that bring you joy and try to incorporate them into your daily routine.
- Take 10 minutes each day to do something that makes you happy, such as reading a book or listening to music.

4. Task: Let go of self-judgment.

- Challenge negative self-talk by asking yourself whether you would say the same thing to a friend.
- Practice gratitude by focusing on what you have, rather than what you lack.
- Write down 3 things that you did well each day and reflect on them.

5. Task: Acknowledge your emotions.

- Create a journal to write down your emotions each day and reflect on how they impact you.
- Practice mindfulness by focusing on the present moment and acknowledging your feelings without judgment.
- Try different techniques for managing emotions, such as deep breathing or visualization.

6. Task: Take a break.

- Create a relaxing environment, such as a cozy nook or a quiet room, where you can retreat to when you need a break.
- Take a 5-minute break every hour to stretch, meditate, or do deep breathing exercises.
- Plan a relaxing activity for yourself, such as a hike or a spa day, for the end of each week.

7. Task: Connect with others.

- Reach out to a friend or family member every day to check in and have a conversation.
- Participate in a support group or join a community to connect with others who have similar experiences.
- Schedule a therapy session with a mental health professional to discuss any challenges or concerns you may have.

Developing a Positive Mindset

Developing a positive mindset is an essential step towards successful weight loss. This is because losing weight and maintaining a healthy weight is not just about what you eat, but it's also about how you think and feel about yourself, food, and your body. A positive and confident mindset will help you make healthier choices, stick to your weight loss plan, and avoid self-sabotage. In this chapter, you will learn how to develop a "skinny mindset" that will support your weight loss journey.

Practice gratitude and self-affirmation.

Point 1 of developing a positive mindset for weight loss is to practice gratitude and self-affirmation. Gratitude and self-affirmation are powerful tools that can help you cultivate a positive mindset and boost your self-esteem.

Gratitude helps you focus on the positive things in your life, rather than dwelling on the negative. By taking a moment each day to reflect on the things you are grateful for, you can cultivate a more positive outlook on life. This positive outlook can spill over into your weight loss journey and help you focus on the progress you are making, rather than dwelling on the setbacks.

Self-affirmation, on the other hand, involves repeating positive statements to yourself. These positive statements can help boost your self-esteem and counteract negative self-talk. Some examples of self-affirmations for weight loss include "I am capable of reaching my weight loss goals," "I am worthy of a healthy body," and "I am strong and determined." Repeat these affirmations to yourself throughout the day, especially when you are feeling discouraged or tempted to give up.

It is also helpful to write down your affirmations and place them in a visible place, such as on your bathroom mirror or in your wallet. Seeing them every day will help reinforce the positive thoughts and beliefs you are trying to cultivate.

In conclusion, practicing gratitude and self-affirmation is an effective way to develop a positive mindset for weight loss. By focusing on the positive things in your life and repeating positive statements to yourself, you can boost your self-esteem, stay motivated, and reach your weight loss goals with a positive and confident attitude.

Here is a gratitude and self-affirmation workbook exercise that you can use to develop a positive mindset for weight loss:

1. Gratitude Journal: Start each day by writing down three things you are grateful for. This can be something as simple as having a roof over your head, a healthy body, or a loving family. Focus on the positive things in your life and let this gratitude spill over into

2. Self-Affirmation Statements: Write down a list of self-affirmation statements that you can repeat to yourself throughout the day. Examples include: "I am capable of reaching my weight loss goals," "I am worthy of a healthy body," "I am strong and determined," "I am proud of myself for trying," etc. Choose affirmations that resonate with you and your weight loss goals.

3. Track Progress: At the end of each week, reflect on your progress and write down any positive changes you have noticed in your mindset. Celebrate the small victories, such as drinking more water or eating a healthy meal, and acknowledge your progress towards your weight loss goals.

4. Reflection: At the end of the month/week, reflect on how your gratitude and self-affirmation practices have impacted your weight loss journey. Have you noticed any positive changes in your mindset? Have you been more motivated and confident in reaching your weight loss goals?

Surround yourself with positive influences.

It's true that the people you surround yourself with can have a big impact on your mindset and success in reaching your weight loss goals. When you're surrounded by positive and supportive individuals, you're more likely to feel encouraged and motivated to stay on track with your journey. These people can provide you with encouragement, accountability, and a sense of community, all of which can help keep you focused and motivated.

On the other hand, exposure to negative influences can have a detrimental effect on your progress. Friends who criticize your weight loss efforts or make unhealthy food choices can be demotivating and discourage you from pursuing your goals. This kind of negativity can also lead to self-doubt and low self-esteem, which can make it difficult for you to stay focused and committed to your journey.

It's important to keep in mind that the people you surround yourself with can influence not only your mindset, but also your behavior. For example, if you're around friends who make unhealthy food choices, you may be more likely to make those same choices yourself. On the other hand, if you're around friends who lead active and healthy lifestyles, you may be more likely to adopt those habits yourself.

So, in order to be successful in your weight loss journey, it's important to surround yourself with positive and supportive people who believe in you and your goals. Surrounding yourself with these individuals can help you stay motivated, focused, and committed to your journey, and can increase your chances of success.

Focus on progress, not perfection.

Perfectionism is a common personality trait that can be both a blessing and a curse. On the one hand, it can drive individuals to strive for excellence and reach their full potential. On the other hand, perfectionism can also become a major barrier to weight loss.

When it comes to weight loss, perfectionism can lead to unrealistic expectations and an all-or-nothing mentality. People with perfectionistic tendencies may set high standards for themselves and become discouraged when they do not see immediate results. They may view any slip-up as a failure and become discouraged, leading to a cycle of self-criticism and discouragement.

This kind of thinking can be particularly harmful when it comes to weight loss, as it ignores the fact that weight loss is a gradual process that takes time and effort. Instead of focusing on being perfect, it is important to focus on making progress towards your weight loss goals.

To overcome perfectionism in weight loss, it is important to celebrate small victories along the way. This could mean acknowledging and congratulating yourself for drinking more water or eating a healthy meal. Celebrating these small successes will help to build confidence and motivation, which can then be harnessed to achieve larger goals.

It is also important to adopt a growth mindset and embrace the concept of progress over perfection. This means focusing on the journey, rather than just the end goal. By focusing on the steps taken towards weight loss, rather than the end result, individuals can better appreciate their efforts and avoid becoming discouraged by setbacks.

Rather than viewing these setbacks as failures, it is important to view them as opportunities to learn and grow.

In conclusion, perfectionism can be a major barrier to weight loss, but it does not have to be. By focusing on progress and celebrating small victories, individuals can overcome perfectionism and achieve their weight loss goals. Remember, the journey to a healthier you is just that—a journey—and it is important to be kind to yourself and embrace progress over perfection.

Exercise: Overcoming Perfectionism in Weight Loss

1. Reflect on your own perfectionistic tendencies and how they may be impacting your weight loss journey.

2. Write down your current weight loss goals.

3. Reframe your goals to focus on progress instead of perfection. For example, instead of "losing 10 pounds in 1 month," try "making healthier food choices and increasing physical activity each week."

4. Write down 3 small victories you have achieved towards your weight loss goals.

5. Write a short paragraph acknowledging and congratulating yourself for each victory.

6. Reflect on any setbacks or slip-ups in your weight loss journey. Write down how you can view these as opportunities to learn and grow, rather than failures.

7. Review your reframed goals and small victories regularly to maintain a growth mindset and stay motivated in your weight loss journey.

By focusing on progress and celebrating small victories, individuals can overcome perfectionism and achieve their weight loss goals. Remember, the journey to a healthier you is just that—a journey—and it is important to be kind to yourself and embrace progress over perfection.

Reframe negative thoughts.

Negative self-talk can be a major obstacle to weight loss. It can be easy to fall into the trap of self-criticism and negativity, especially when progress seems slow or setbacks arise. However, these negative thoughts can have a major impact on our motivation and determination to stick to our weight loss goals.

When negative thoughts arise, it is important to take a moment to stop and reframe them. Instead of thinking "I can't stick to my diet," think "I am making progress and I am proud of myself for trying." This small shift in perspective can help us maintain a positive mindset and stay motivated.

It is also important to remember that weight loss is a journey, not a destination. There will be ups and downs, and it is normal to have setbacks along the way. But, with a positive attitude and the determination to keep trying, we can overcome these obstacles and reach our goals.

One effective way to reframe negative thoughts is to practice gratitude. Take a moment to think about all of the things in your life that you are grateful for, and focus on these positive aspects instead of dwelling on negative thoughts. This can help shift your perspective and keep you motivated.

Another technique to try is visualization. Imagine yourself reaching your weight loss goals and picture yourself feeling proud and confident. Visualizing positive outcomes can help you stay focused on your goals and maintain a positive attitude.

It is also helpful to seek support from others. Surround yourself with positive, supportive people who encourage you and believe in your abilities. Talking to a trusted friend or family member about your weight loss journey can also help you gain a fresh perspective and reframe negative thoughts.

In conclusion, negative self-talk can be a major obstacle to weight loss. However, with the right tools and techniques, we can overcome this challenge and maintain a positive mindset.

Remember to take a moment to reframe negative thoughts, practice gratitude, visualize positive outcomes, and seek support from others. With these strategies in place, you can stay motivated and achieve your weight loss goals.

Exercise: Reframing Negative Thoughts for Weight Loss Success

This exercise will help you identify and reframe negative thoughts that may be hindering your progress towards your weight loss goals.

Step 1: Write down any negative thoughts that come to mind when you think about your weight loss journey. Examples may include: "I'll never be able to stick to my diet," "I'm too weak to resist temptations," or "I'll never reach my goal weight."

Step 2: For each negative thought, write down a reframed, positive thought. Use the format "Instead of thinking 'I'll never be able to stick to my diet,' I will think 'I am making progress and I am proud of myself for trying.'"

Step 3: Reflect on why these negative thoughts may be coming up for you. Are they based on past experiences? Do they stem from self-doubt or insecurity? Understanding the root cause of your negative thoughts can help you address them more effectively.

Step 4: Use visualization and gratitude to further shift your perspective. Visualize yourself reaching your weight loss goals and feeling proud and confident. Write it down. Practice gratitude by taking time each day to think about all of the things in your life and about your body right now that you are grateful for.

Step 5: Practice reframing negative thoughts in real-time. Whenever you catch yourself having a negative thought, stop and reframe it in a positive light. Over time, this will become a habit and will help you maintain a positive mindset.

Step 6: Seek support from others. Talk to a trusted friend or family member about your weight loss journey and seek encouragement and support from positive, supportive people in your life.

By completing this exercise, you will have taken an important step towards overcoming negative self-talk and staying motivated on your weight loss journey. Remember, with the right tools and techniques, you can achieve your goals and feel proud of your progress along the way.

Practice mindfulness.

Mindfulness is a simple but powerful practice that can help us cultivate a healthier and more balanced life. It involves being present in the moment and paying attention to our thoughts, feelings, and sensations without judgment. By doing so, mindfulness can help us better understand our bodies and emotions, making it easier to avoid overeating and emotional eating. In this chapter, we will explore the benefits of mindfulness, how it can help us achieve a healthy lifestyle, and simple mindfulness techniques that anyone can try.

The Benefits of Mindfulness

Mindfulness has been shown to have a variety of positive effects on our mental and physical well-being. Research has found that mindfulness can reduce stress and anxiety, lower blood pressure, and improve sleep quality. It can also help us tune into our body's hunger and fullness signals, making it easier to avoid overeating. Additionally, mindfulness has been shown to reduce symptoms of depression and improve overall mood.

Mindfulness and a Healthy Lifestyle

One of the biggest benefits of mindfulness is that it can help us achieve a healthier lifestyle. When we are mindful, we are more aware of our eating habits, including when and why we eat. This awareness can help us avoid overeating and make healthier food choices. Additionally, mindfulness can help us reduce stress and anxiety, which can lead to emotional eating. By practicing mindfulness, we can cultivate a positive and relaxed mindset, which can have a ripple effect on all aspects of our lives.

There are many different mindfulness techniques that you can try, including deep breathing, meditation, and yoga. One simple mindfulness technique is deep breathing. To practice deep breathing, simply find a quiet place to sit and focus on your breath. Take a deep breath in, hold it for a few seconds, and then slowly exhale. Repeat this process for several minutes, focusing solely on your breath.

Meditation is another mindfulness technique that can help you cultivate a relaxed and peaceful state of mind. To practice meditation, find a quiet place to sit and focus on your breath. You can also use guided meditations or guided imagery exercises to help you relax and focus.

Finally, yoga is a mindfulness technique that combines physical movement and breath control. By practicing yoga, you can develop greater body awareness, reduce stress and anxiety, and cultivate a positive and relaxed mindset.

In conclusion, mindfulness is a powerful tool that can help us achieve a healthier and more balanced life. Whether it's through deep breathing, meditation, or yoga, the benefits of mindfulness are numerous and far-reaching. So why not give it a try today and start reaping the rewards of a mindful lifestyle?

Mindfulness exercises for achieving a healthy lifestyle:

- **Deep Breathing Exercise:** Find a quiet place to sit and focus on your breath. Take a deep breath in, hold it for a few seconds, and then slowly exhale. Repeat this process for several minutes, focusing solely on your breath.

- **Meditation Exercise:** Find a quiet place to sit and focus on your breath. You can also use guided meditations or guided imagery exercises to help you relax and focus. Start with 5-10 minutes of meditation and gradually increase the time as you become more comfortable with the practice.

- **Yoga Exercise:** Find a yoga class or YouTube video to follow, or simply practice simple yoga poses at home. Focus on your breath and body movements, and try to cultivate a sense of peace and relaxation.

- **Body Scan Exercise:** Lie down on your back with your eyes closed. Starting from your toes, focus on each part of your body, noticing any sensations or feelings. Move slowly up your body, paying attention to each part until you reach the top of your head.

- **Gratitude Exercise:** Take a few minutes each day to reflect on what you are grateful for. Write down a list of things you are grateful for or simply reflect on them in your mind. This exercise can help you cultivate a positive and grateful mindset.

- **Body Awareness Exercise:** Take a few minutes each day to simply focus on your body. Notice how your clothes feel against your skin, the sensations in your feet, and any other feelings or sensations. This exercise can help you tune into your body's hunger and fullness signals and reduce emotional eating.

By incorporating these mindfulness exercises into your daily routine, you can start to experience the benefits of mindfulness, including reduced stress and anxiety, improved mood, and a healthier lifestyle.

Space for your thoughts:

Embrace your body and treat it with love and respect.

One of the most important steps towards developing a positive mindset is embracing your body and treating it with love and respect. Instead of criticizing your body or comparing yourself to others, focus on the things you love about yourself and your body.

Many people struggle with body image and low self-esteem due to societal standards and media representation of beauty. It's easy to get caught up in criticism and comparison, but these negative thoughts only serve to harm our self-worth and happiness. Instead of focusing on what's wrong with our bodies, we need to concentrate on our unique strengths and qualities. By celebrating our bodies for what they can do, rather than what they look like, we can cultivate a sense of self-worth that leads to greater happiness and confidence.

One effective way to embrace your body is to focus on your abilities. Your body is capable of incredible things, from supporting you in your daily activities to helping you reach your goals and dreams. Take a moment to think about all the amazing things your body can do, from the simple act of breathing to more complex movements like running or playing an instrument. By focusing on these abilities, you can shift your focus from physical appearance to the many ways your body supports you every day.

Another important step in embracing your body is to take care of it. This means treating it with love and respect, and nourishing it with healthy food and regular exercise. Regular exercise is not only good for your physical health, but it also boosts your mood and helps reduce stress. Eating nutritious food and staying hydrated can also have a positive impact on your body and mind.

Workbook Exercise: Embracing Your Body

Objective: To help you develop a positive mindset and embrace your body through self-reflection and goal-setting.

Instructions:
1. Reflect on your current relationship with your body. Write down your thoughts, feelings, and beliefs about your body, both positive and negative.

2. Identify specific areas of your body that you struggle to embrace. Write down why these areas are difficult for you, and how you can work on changing your negative thoughts about them.

Developing a Positive Mindset

3. Focus on your body's abilities. Write down a list of everything your body can do, both big and small. Examples might include walking, running, playing an instrument, or simply breathing.

4. Celebrate your strengths. Write down a list of qualities that make you unique and special, focusing on both physical and non-physical traits. Remember, your worth is not determined by your appearance.

5. Create a self-care plan. Write down steps you can take to take care of your body, such as exercising regularly, eating nutritious food, getting enough sleep, and practicing self-care rituals.

6. Set achievable goals. Write down a few specific, achievable goals related to embracing your body and developing a positive mindset. Examples might include practicing self-love affirmations every day, or taking a dance class to focus on your body's abilities.

7. Reflection. Write down your thoughts and feelings about this exercise, and what you learned about your relationship with your body.

8. Repeat these exercises regularly to continue to build a positive relationship with your body and cultivate a sense of self-worth and happiness.

Remember, embracing your body and developing a positive mindset takes time and effort, but the rewards are worth it. By focusing on your strengths and abilities, treating your body with love and respect, and setting achievable goals, you can create a healthier, happier life for yourself.

Developing a positive mindset is a critical step towards successful weight loss. By practicing gratitude, self-affirmation, mind-fulness, and embracing your body, you can cultivate a "skinny mindset" that will support you on your weight loss journey. Remember to be kind and patient with yourself, and focus on progress, not perfection. With time, effort, and a positive mindset, you will be able to reach your weight loss goals and maintain a healthy weight for life.

Setting Weight Loss Goals

Weight loss can be a challenging journey, and many people often struggle to stick to their diet and exercise regimen. Setting weight loss goals can help you stay motivated and focused on your path to a healthier lifestyle. In this chapter, we will discuss why setting weight loss goals is important and how it can help you achieve success.

1. **Clarity and Direction:** When you set a weight loss goal, you have a clear direction of where you want to go and what you want to achieve. This clarity helps you prioritize your efforts and make decisions that support your goal. It also gives you a sense of purpose and direction, making it easier to stay motivated.

2. **Measurable Progress:** When you set weight loss goals, you can track your progress and measure your success. This tracking process helps you to stay accountable and see the results of your efforts. It can also provide encouragement and a sense of accomplishment, which can further motivate you to keep going.

3. **Realistic Expectations:** Setting realistic weight loss goals helps you avoid disappointment and frustration. If you set achievable goals, you are more likely to stick to your diet and exercise regimen, and you can experience the benefits of weight loss without getting discouraged.

4. **Flexibility:** Setting weight loss goals also provides flexibility, as you can adjust your goals as needed. For example, if you find that you are losing weight slower than you anticipated, you can adjust your goal to reflect a more realistic timeline. This flexibility helps you stay motivated and avoid giving up on your weight loss journey.

5. **Long-Term Success:** Weight loss is a long-term process, and setting goals can help you achieve long-term success. When you set a goal, you are committing to making a change in your lifestyle and creating a plan for how you will maintain your weight loss over time. This long-term perspective helps you stay focused and motivated, even when faced with challenges.

In conclusion, setting weight loss goals is an important part of the weight loss journey. It provides clarity, direction, and a sense of purpose, which can help you stay motivated and achieve success. Whether you are just starting your weight loss journey or are looking to take it to the next level, setting goals can help you reach your desired outcome and maintain a healthier lifestyle.

Determine Your Starting Point

Before you can set your weight loss goals, it's important to deter-mine where you're starting from. This means taking an accurate measurement of your current weight, body fat percentage, and waist circumference. It's also helpful to keep a food diary for a few days, to get a sense of your current eating habits.

Current weight:

Body Fat percentage:

Waist circumference:

Identify Your Reasons for Wanting to Lose Weight
Why do you want to lose weight? Is it to improve your health? To fit into a specific outfit? To increase your energy levels? Identifying your reasons for wanting to lose weight will help you stay motivated, as you'll have a clear understanding of what you're working towards.

Set Realistic and Specific Goals

When setting your weight loss goals, it's important to be realistic. Aiming to lose 10 pounds in a week is not only unrealistic, but it's also not sustainable. A healthy rate of weight loss is between 1-2 pounds per week. Setting specific goals, such as "I want to lose 10 pounds in the next 3 months" or "I want to reduce my body fat percentage by 5% in 6 months," will help you stay focused and motivated.

Make Your Goals Measurable

To ensure that you're on track to achieving your goals, it's important to make them measurable. For example, instead of simply saying "I want to eat healthier," you could say "I want to eat at least 5 servings of fruits and vegetables every day." Measurable goals allow you to track your progress, and make adjustments to your plan as needed.

Create a Plan of Action

Once you have set your weight loss goals, it's time to create a plan of action. This might include a specific exercise routine, a healthy eating plan, and strategies for overcoming obstacles that might arise. Having a plan in place will help you stay focused and motivated, and ensure that you're on track to achieving your goals.

Letting Go of Dieting and Embracing Intuitive Eating

Letting go of dieting and embracing intuitive eating is a journey that can be both challenging and liberating. Dieting often involves restrictive eating patterns and a focus on external measures of success, such as weight loss or body size. In contrast, intuitive eating is an approach that emphasizes listening to your body's natural hunger and fullness cues, and allowing yourself to eat what you truly want and need, without judgment or guilt. This shift can be difficult, especially if you've spent a long time trying to control your eating and body size, but it can lead to greater happiness and health in the long run.

The first step in letting go of dieting and embracing intuitive eating is to question your beliefs about food and your body. Many people who have dieted for a long time have internalized a set of rules about what is "good" and "bad" food, and what their ideal body size and shape should be. These beliefs can be deeply ingrained, and can be difficult to challenge. However, it's important to question whether these beliefs are truly serving you and your health, or whether they are holding you back from enjoying life and feeling good in your own skin.

Once you've questioned your beliefs, it's time to start listening to your body. This may mean allowing yourself to eat what you truly want, without restriction, and without trying to control your portions. It may also mean allowing yourself to eat larger portions if you're truly hungry, and stopping eating when you're full, even if there is still food on your plate. The key is to listen to your body's natural hunger and fullness cues, and to eat in a way that feels good and satisfying.

It's also important to be mindful of the emotional reasons why you may be reaching for food. Sometimes, people use food as a way to cope with stress, anxiety, or other emotions. While there is nothing inherently wrong with this, it's important to be aware of what is driving your food choices, and to seek alternative ways to cope with your emotions. For example, you may find that going for a walk or practicing mindfulness is a more effective way to manage your stress than reaching for food.

In addition to listening to your body, it's important to cultivate a positive relationship with food. This means learning to enjoy food for its own sake, rather than just for its nutritional value or for the way it makes you look. This may involve trying new foods, cooking for yourself, or eating in a more relaxed and enjoyable environment.

Finally, it's important to be patient with yourself as you make this transition. Letting go of dieting and embracing intuitive eating is a journey, and it may take time to fully break free from old habits and patterns. However, with patience and persistence, you will learn to trust your body, and to enjoy food and your body in a new and more positive way.

1. Reflecting on Your Thoughts and Beliefs about Food and Your Body:
   - Write down your current thoughts and beliefs about food and your body. What are your "rules" about what is "good" and "bad" food? What do you believe your ideal body size and shape should be?

- Reflect on whether these beliefs are truly serving you and your health. What would happen if you let go of these beliefs and allowed yourself to listen to your body's natural hunger and fullness cues?

2. Practicing Mindful Eating:

- Choose one meal to focus on this week. Set aside any distractions (such as phones, books, or televisions) and focus solely on your food.
- Pay attention to your body's hunger and fullness cues. How does your body feel before you start eating? How does it feel as you eat? How does it feel after you finish eating?

- Try to savor each bite of food, paying attention to its taste, texture, and smell. What do you enjoy about this food?

- After the meal, reflect on your experience. Did you feel more satisfied and connected to your food?

1. Identifying Your Emotional Eating Triggers:

- Keep a food diary for one week, noting what you eat, how much you eat, and how you feel before, during, and after eating(you can food diary templates at the end of the book).

- Look for patterns in your food choices. Are there certain times or situations when you tend to eat more or eat differently?

- Consider what emotions or stressors may be driving your food choices. Are you using food as a way to cope with stress, boredom, or other emotions?

Once you've identified your emotional eating triggers, try to find alternative ways to cope with these emotions. For example, you may try going for a walk, practicing mindfulness, or reaching out to a friend.

Space for your thoughts:

Cultivating a Positive Relationship with Food:

- Try one new food this week. Choose something that you've never tried before, or something that you've been avoiding.

- Cook a meal for yourself or a loved one. Take the time to choose ingredients, prepare the food, and enjoy the process.

- Eat in a relaxed and enjoyable environment, free from distractions. This could mean eating a meal with friends, eating outside in nature, or simply eating at a slower pace.

- After each of these experiences, reflect on how it made you feel. Did you enjoy the food more? Did you feel more positive about your relationship with food?

Being Patient and Compassionate with Yourself:

- Remember that letting go of dieting and embracing intuitive eating is a journey, and it may take time to fully break free from old habits and patterns.

- Practice self-compassion. Treat yourself with the same kindness and understanding that you would offer to a close friend.

- Celebrate your successes, no matter how small they may seem. Recognize the progress you have made and remind yourself of why this journey is important to you.

By working through these exercises, you will begin to develop a healthier and more positive relationship with food and your body. Remember to be patient with yourself and to celebrate your progress, no matter how small it may seem. With time and persistence, you will learn to trust your body and to enjoy food in a new and more positive way.

Cultivating Gratitude and Positive Body Image

Cultivating gratitude is one of the most important tools that you can use in your journey towards weight loss and positive body image. This simple yet powerful practice has been shown to have a profound impact on our overall health and wellbeing, and can help to foster a more positive and empowered outlook on life.

One of the key benefits of cultivating gratitude is that it helps us to shift our focus away from our negative thoughts and experiences, and towards the things that we are thankful for. This can be incredibly important in the context of weight loss and positive body image, as it can help to reduce feelings of stress, anxiety, and self-criticism that often arise when we are trying to make changes in these areas of our lives. By focusing on the things that we are grateful for, we can reduce the negative self-talk that often accompanies our thoughts about our bodies, and instead cultivate a more positive and uplifting outlook.

In addition to reducing negative self-talk, cultivating gratitude can also help to foster a more positive body image. This is because gratitude encourages us to focus on our strengths and the things that we love about ourselves, rather than our perceived flaws and weaknesses. By embracing gratitude and focusing on the things that we are proud of, we can start to feel more confident in our own skin, and develop a more positive and empowering relationship with our bodies.

Another important benefit of cultivating gratitude is that it can help to foster a healthier relationship with food. Gratitude helps us to cultivate a more mindful and present approach to eating, as we become more aware of the positive experiences and feelings that come with nourishing our bodies with healthy food. This can help to reduce the negative associations that often accompany our thoughts about food, and instead encourage us to view food as a source of energy, nourishment, and enjoyment.

Finally, cultivating gratitude is also a powerful tool for weight loss. This is because gratitude encourages us to be more mindful of our eating habits, and helps us to make more informed decisions about the foods that we eat. By taking a more intentional and mindful approach to eating, we can reduce the likelihood of overeating and making unhealthy food choices, and instead focus on nourishing our bodies with healthy, whole foods that provide us with the energy and nutrients that we need to be healthy and thrive.

Here are some workbook exercises to help you cultivate gratitude and improve your weight loss and positive body image journey. These will also help to reinforce habits established earlier in the book:

Gratitude journaling: Take some time each day to write down three things that you are grateful for. This could be something as simple as a beautiful sunset, a delicious meal, or a kind act from someone in your life. Writing down what you are grateful for helps to shift your focus away from negative thoughts and towards the positive aspects of your life.

Positive affirmations: Write down positive affirmations that focus on your strengths, accomplishments, and the things that you love about yourself. Read these affirmations to yourself each morning, and throughout the day as needed, to help reinforce a positive and empowered outlook on your body image.

Body appreciation: Focus on and write down the things that you love about your body. This could be something as simple as appreciating your strong legs, or the way your hair shines in the sun. By focusing on the things that you love about your body, you can start to develop a more positive and empowered relationship with it.

Gratitude walks: Take a walk outside and focus on the things that you are grateful for in your environment. This could be anything from the trees swaying in the wind, to the sound of birds singing, or the feel of the sun on your skin. By taking the time to focus on the things that you are grateful for, you can reduce stress and anxiety, and cultivate a more positive outlook on life.

Overcoming Emotional Eating and Cravings

Emotional eating and cravings can be difficult to manage, but with the right strategies and tools, they can be overcome. Here are some effective ways to overcome emotional eating and cravings:

Identify the root cause of your cravings: Understanding why you turn to food for comfort can help you develop a plan to manage it. Try to identify your root cause for emotional eating. That can occur for variety of reasons:

Stress: Stressful situations can trigger feelings of anxiety, depression, or frustration, which can lead to cravings for high-fat, high-sugar, or high-carbohydrate foods.

Boredom: Boredom can lead to mindless snacking, which can quickly add up to a significant amount of calories.

Loneliness: Loneliness can trigger cravings for comfort foods that bring back happy memories or provide a temporary sense of comfort.

Hormonal imbalances: Hormonal changes, such as those that occur during menstrual cycles or menopause, can lead to cravings for certain types of foods, such as sugar or carbs.

Past experiences: Childhood experiences, such as being offered food as a reward or being comforted with food during difficult times, can lead to emotional eating in adulthood.

Lack of sleep: Lack of sleep can lead to hormonal imbalances that trigger cravings for high-calorie, high-fat, or high-sugar foods.

Environmental cues: Certain sights, smells, or sounds can trigger cravings, especially if they are associated with a positive experience or emotion.

Practice mindfulness: By focusing on the present moment, you can learn to identify and manage your cravings without turning to food. Practicing mindfulness during emotional eating and cravings can help you become more aware of your thoughts, feelings, and bodily sensations. Here are some steps to practice mindfulness during these moments:

1. Pause: When you feel the urge to emotionally eat, take a moment to pause and become aware of your thoughts and feelings. Don't judge yourself for having cravings, but simply acknowledge them.

2. Check in with your body: Pay attention to any physical sensations you're experiencing, such as hunger, thirst, or discomfort. Try to identify what your body truly needs.

3. Practice deep breathing: Take a few deep breaths, inhaling deeply and exhaling slowly, to help calm your mind and body. This can help you become more present and mindful in the moment.

4. Label your thoughts and emotions: Try to identify and label the thoughts and emotions you're experiencing. For example, you might say to yourself, "I'm feeling stressed right now," or "I'm craving something sweet."

5. Choose a healthy response: Once you've become more aware of your thoughts and feelings, choose a healthy response to manage your cravings. This could include taking a walk, drinking water, or finding a healthier alternative to the food you're craving.

6. Focus on the present moment: Instead of dwelling on the past or worrying about the future, focus on the present moment. Pay attention to your surroundings and the sensations you're experiencing, such as the sounds, smells, and textures of the food you're eating.

By practicing mindfulness during emotional eating and cravings, you can become more aware of your thoughts and feelings and make healthier choices. Over time, this can help you develop a healthier relationship with food and reduce the frequency and intensity of your cravings.

The Importance of Mindful Eating

Mindful eating is a concept that has gained popularity in recent years as a means of promoting better health and wellness. It involves paying attention to your food, the act of eating, and your body's physical and emotional responses to food. This approach to eating is based on the idea that our relationship with food can have a significant impact on our overall well-being, both physically and mentally. In this chapter, we will explore the importance of mindful eating and how it can benefit individuals in their daily lives.

One of the key benefits of mindful eating is improved digestion. When we eat mindfully, we are able to fully focus on the food we are consuming, which allows us to chew our food thoroughly. This helps to break down the food in our mouths, making it easier for our digestive system to process. Additionally, when we eat mindfully, we are less likely to eat too quickly, which can lead to indigestion and discomfort.

Another important benefit of mindful eating is a reduction in overeating. Many people struggle with overeating, either due to emotional reasons or simply because they are not paying attention to their body's signals of hunger and fullness. Mindful eating encourages individuals to tune into their bodies, to recognize the physical sensations of hunger and fullness, and to respond accordingly. This helps to prevent overeating and to maintain a healthy weight.

Mindful eating can also have a positive impact on our mental health. Eating is often associated with stress, anxiety, and negative emotions. By focusing on the act of eating, individuals can learn to calm their minds and reduce stress. Additionally, the act of paying attention to the food we are consuming can help to foster a sense of gratitude and appreciation for the food we have. This, in turn, can help to improve our overall mood and reduce feelings of depression and anxiety.

Another benefit of mindful eating is improved nutrient absorption. When we eat mindfully, we are able to fully savor and enjoy our food, which can help to increase our enjoyment of the meal. This increased enjoyment can lead to better digestion and absorption of nutrients from the food we are consuming. Furthermore, when we eat mindfully, we are less likely to eat foods that are high in processed ingredients, which can decrease the overall quality of our diet. Mindful eating can help to build a healthier relationship with food. Many individuals struggle with disordered eating patterns, such as binge eating, emotional eating, and restrictive eating. Mindful eating encourages individuals to focus on their food and their bodies, rather than on their emotions or external factors. This can help to break negative patterns and promote a healthier relationship with food.

In conclusion, mindful eating is a valuable tool for promoting better health and wellness. By paying attention to our food, the act of eating, and our body's physical and emotional responses to food, individuals can improve their digestion, reduce overeating, improve their mental health, increase nutrient absorption, and build a healthier relationship with food. Whether you are looking to improve your overall well-being or simply to enjoy your food more fully, incorporating mindful eating into your daily routine can be a beneficial and transformative experience.

How to Practice Mindful Eating and Movement

Mindful eating is a practice that involves paying attention to the sensations and experiences of eating. This includes paying attention to hunger and fullness signals, savoring the flavors and textures of food, and being present in the moment while eating. The goal of mindful eating is to increase awareness and enjoyment of food, while also reducing stress and overeating.

How to Practice Mindful Eating

1. Start by creating a peaceful environment. Find a quiet place to sit down, free from distractions, and take a few deep breaths to relax.

2. Pay attention to your hunger levels. Before you begin eating, take a moment to assess your hunger levels. Are you starving, or just feeling a little peckish? This will help you determine how much food you need to eat.

3. Serve yourself a reasonable portion. Avoid overeating by serving yourself a reasonable portion of food on your plate.

4. Slow down and savor your food. Chew your food slowly and deliberately, taking the time to taste and appreciate each bite. Avoid distractions like watching TV or using your phone while eating.

5. Pay attention to fullness signals. As you eat, pay attention to your body's signals of fullness. Stop eating when you feel satisfied, rather than stuffed.

6. Reflect on your eating experience. After you finish eating, take a few minutes to reflect on your experience. What did you enjoy about the meal? What could have been better? This will help you make healthier choices in the future.

What is Mindful Movement?

Mindful movement is a practice that involves paying attention to your body and the sensations it experiences during physical activity. This includes paying attention to your breathing, posture, and movements, and being present in the moment while moving. The goal of mindful movement is to increase awareness and enjoyment of physical activity, while also reducing stress and promoting better health.

How to Practice Mindful Movement

- Choose an activity that you enjoy. Find a physical activity that youenjoy, whether it's yoga, walking, or dancing. The key is to choose something that you find enjoyable and that you'll look forward to doing.

- Start slowly. Begin with a gentle warm-up, such as stretching or light cardio. This will help you get into the right mindset and prepare your body for the activity.

- Pay attention to your breathing. Throughout the activity, focus on your breathing and make sure you're taking deep, slow breaths.

- Pay attention to your posture. Stand tall and maintain good posture throughout the activity. This will help you avoid injury and get the most out of the activity.

- Pay attention to your movements. Focus on your movements and the sensations in your body as you move. Try to be present in the moment and avoid distractions like listening to music or watching TV.

- Reflect on your experience. After you finish the activity, take a few minutes to reflect on your experience. What did you enjoy about the activity? What could have been better? This will help you make healthier choices in the future.

Developing a Growth Mindset

A growth mindset is a powerful tool for personal and professional development. It is based on the idea that we have the ability to grow and develop, and that our abilities, intelligence, and characteristics are not fixed but can be shaped and moulded through effort and learning. This approach to life is empowering and encourages individuals to take risks, embrace challenges, and continue to learn and grow.

People with a growth mindset believe that they can improve and develop their skills and abilities, and are more likely to engage in activities that challenge them. This can lead to greater motivation, as individuals are more likely to seek out opportunities for growth and development. This mindset also leads to greater resilience, as individuals are less likely to give up when faced with obstacles or failures. Instead, they see these challenges as opportunities to learn and grow.

In a professional setting, a growth mindset can be particularly valuable. Those with a growth mindset are more likely to be proactive in their work, seeking out new opportunities for learning and development. They are also more likely to embrace change, viewing it as an opportu-nity for growth rather than a threat. This mindset can lead to greater innovation, as individuals are more likely to take risks and experiment with new ideas.

In contrast, a fixed mindset can hold individuals back, as they believe that their abilities and characteristics are set in stone and cannot be changed. This approach can lead to a lack of motivation, as individuals do not see the point in taking risks or engaging in challenging activities. It can also lead to a lack of resilience, as individuals may be more likely to give up when faced with obstacles or failures.

The idea of a growth mindset is highly relevant to losing weight and keeping it off. This is because weight loss and maintenance require a significant amount of effort and learning, and individuals must be willing to continuously develop and improve their habits and behaviours.

A growth mindset can help individuals approach weight loss as a journey of growth and development, rather than a one-time event. This mindset encourages individuals to embrace challenges and overcome obstacles, and to view failures as opportunities to learn and grow. This approach can lead to greater motivation and resilience, as individuals are more likely to stay committed to their weight loss goals, even when faced with setbacks.

Additionally, a growth mindset can help individuals develop a positive relationship with food and their bodies. Rather than viewing weight loss as a punishment or restriction, individuals with a growth mindset may view it as an opportunity to learn about healthy eating habits and develop a healthy relationship with food. This approach can lead to greater success in maintaining weight loss, as individuals are more likely to adopt healthy habits that are sustainable over the long term.

How to Develop a Growth Mindset

1. Practice Self-Reflection

Take time each day to reflect on your thoughts and behaviors. Ask yourself how you can improve and what steps you can take to reach your goals. This can help you identify negative thought patterns and replace them with more positive and constructive ones.

2. Embrace Challenges

Challenges are opportunities to learn and grow. Embracing them, rather than avoiding them, can help you develop a growth mindset. When faced with a difficult task, try to see it as an opportunity to learn and improve, rather than as a threat to your abilities.

3. Celebrate Progress

Celebrate small victories along the way to your goals. This will help you stay motivated and see the progress you are making, even if it is slow. This can also help you develop a more positive self-image and build your confidence.

4. Focus on the Process

Instead of fixating on the end result, focus on the process of achieving your goals. This can help you stay motivated and enjoy the journey, rather than becoming discouraged by setbacks or slow progress.

5. Surround Yourself with Positive Influences

Surround yourself with people who support and encourage you. Seek out individuals who have a growth mindset and who will help you stay motivated and focused on your goals.

Staying Committed to the Skinny Mindset with a Growth Mindset

Set Realistic Goals

Setting achievable and realistic goals is an important aspect of maintaining a healthy and positive mindset. It helps you to stay focused and motivated, while also allowing you to measure your progress and see the results of your efforts. By setting achievable goals, you can avoid feeling overwhelmed or discouraged, and instead, feel a sense of accomplishment and satisfaction as you work towards your desired outcome.

When setting your goals, it is important to keep them realistic and aligned with your current lifestyle and capabilities. This means considering factors such as your schedule, responsibilities, and personal limitations. For example, if you are trying to adopt a healthier eating habit, starting by incorporating more fruits and vegetables into your meals, rather than trying to completely overhaul your diet overnight, is a more achievable and realistic goal.

It is also important to focus on progress, rather than perfection. No one is perfect, and it is okay to make mistakes along the way. The important thing is to learn from those mistakes, and to keep moving forward. Celebrate small victories and progress, no matter how small they may seem, as they can be powerful motivators to keep you going.

By setting achievable and realistic goals and focusing on progress, rather than perfection, you can maintain a positive and sustainable skinny mindset. This will help you to stay committed to your goals, and to make lasting changes that will improve your overall health and well-being.

Goal-Setting Exercise

Step 1: Reflect on your current habits and lifestyle

- Take some time to reflect on your current habits and lifestyle, and think about what changes you would like to make in order to achieve a healthy and positive mindset.

Step 2: Identify your goals

- Write down your goals in a clear and specific manner, making sure they are achievable and realistic.
- For example, instead of saying "I want to eat healthier," say "I want to incorporate more fruits and vegetables into my meals."

Step 3: Break down your goals into smaller, achievable tasks

- For each goal, break it down into smaller, achievable tasks that you can work on over time.
- For example, if your goal is to incorporate more fruits and vegetables into your meals, your first task might be to plan out your meals for the week and make a shopping list of the fruits and vegetables you will need.

Step 4: Prioritize your goals

- Prioritize your goals based on their importance and urgency, and focus on working on the most important ones first.

Step 5: Track your progress

- Keep a journal or a record of your progress, and track your achievements along the way. This will help you to stay motivated and see the results of your efforts.

Step 6: Celebrate your successes

- Celebrate your successes, no matter how small they may seem, as they can be powerful motivators to keep you going.

Step 7: Review and adjust

- Regularly review your progress, and make adjustments to your goals and tasks as needed.

By following these steps, you can set achievable and realistic goals for yourself and maintain a positive and sustainable mindset. Remember to focus on progress, rather than perfection, and to celebrate your successes along the way.

Focus on Healthy Habits

This may sound obvious, yet this is the most proven weigh-loss method known so far - developing healthy habits is crucial in maintaining a "skinny mindset," as it requires a holistic approach to one's health and well-being. Eating a balanced diet is the foundation of a healthy lifestyle, as it provides the body with the essential nutrients it needs to function properly. This means eating a variety of foods from different food groups, and limiting the intake of processed and high-fat foods.

Getting regular exercise is another important aspect of developing healthy habits. Exercise not only helps to maintain a healthy weight, but also provides numerous physical and mental health benefits. Whether it's going for a walk, taking a yoga class, or lifting weights, it's important to find an activity that you enjoy and make it a regular part of your routine.

Self-care is also a critical component of a healthy lifestyle. This includes taking time for yourself to recharge and prioritize your mental and emotional well-being. This can be as simple as reading a book, taking a relaxing bath, or meditating.

It's important to focus on the positive aspects of these habits, such as the improved physical and mental well-being they bring, rather than viewing them as restrictions. This shift in mindset can make it easier to embrace these habits as part of a healthy lifestyle and stay committed to the "skinny mindset." By making healthy habits a priority, you can improve your overall quality of life and achieve and maintain a healthy weight.

Embracing a Healthy Lifestyle Exercise

1. Write down your current eating habits. Be specific and honest with yourself.

2. Identify any areas where you could improve your diet, such as eating more fruits and vegetables or limiting processed foods.

3. Make a list of physical activities that you enjoy. This could be anything from dancing to hiking to playing a sport.

4. Set a goal for incorporating regular exercise into your routine. This could be as simple as going for a walk for 30 minutes a day, or committing to a yoga class once a week.

5. Write down three self-care activities that you can incorporate into your routine. This could be anything from taking a relaxing bath to reading a book before bed.

6. Reflect on the positive aspects of developing healthy habits. Write down how eating a balanced diet, getting regular exercise, and practicing self-care will improve your physical and mental well-being.

7. Create an action plan for incorporating these healthy habits into your daily routine. Be specific and set realistic goals for yourself.

8. Finally, remind yourself that embracing these habits as part of a healthy lifestyle is a positive step towards improved overall health and well-being.

Remember, the key to staying committed to the "skinny mindset" is to focus on the positive aspects of healthy habits and embrace them as part of a healthy lifestyle

Practice Self-Compassion

Self-compassion and kindness towards oneself is a crucial aspect of mental wellness. Negative self-talk can be harmful to your self-esteem and can create a vicious cycle of self-doubt and dissatisfaction. By practicing self-compassion, you can break this cycle and develop a more positive relationship with yourself.

One way to practice self-compassion is by replacing negative self-talk with positive affirmations. This means acknowledging your strengths and accomplishments, and reminding yourself of your worth. It's important to be gentle with yourself and avoid harsh judgment or criticism. Instead, talk to yourself as you would talk to a friend, using words of encouragement and understanding.

Additionally, self-compassion involves recognizing and acknowledging your struggles and difficulties, rather than ignoring or denying them. It's important to be mindful of your emotions and to give yourself permission to feel them, rather than trying to suppress or avoid them. When you approach your experiences with self-compassion, you create a safe and supportive environment for yourself, which can help you to feel more resilient and better equipped to handle life's challenges.

In summary, practicing self-compassion can help you to develop a more positive and healthy relationship with yourself. By being kind and compassionate towards yourself, you can reduce the impact of negative self-talk, build your self-esteem, and create a foundation for overall well-being.

Here is another exercise to develop a more positive and compassionate relationship with yourself, and to reduce the impact of negative self-talk.

1. Take a moment to reflect on your current relationship with yourself. Write down any negative self-talk or criticisms that come to mind.

2. Now, think about the things that you are proud of and the things that you are good at. Write down a list of your strengths and accomplishments.

3. For each item on your list of strengths and accomplishments, write a positive affirmation that celebrates and affirms it. For example, if one of your strengths is that you are a good listener, you could write, "I am a compassionate and attentive listener who makes others feel heard and valued."

- When you catch yourself engaging in negative self-talk, take a moment to pause and challenge that thought. Replace it with one of the positive affirmations from your list.

- Be mindful of your emotions and experiences, and approach them with self-compassion. Allow yourself to feel your emotions, and talk to yourself with kindness and understanding.

- Finally, reflect on your progress and continue to build upon your self-compassion practice. Remember to be patient and gentle with yourself, and celebrate your progress along the way.

Learn from Setbacks

Setbacks are an inevitable and normal part of the process of pursuing a healthy lifestyle. It's common for people to encounter obstacles and challenges along the way, but it's important to not let these setbacks discourage you. Instead of feeling defeated, try to view these setbacks as opportunities for growth and learning. Take a step back and reflect on what you can do differently next time to avoid similar setbacks.

It's important to understand that setbacks are not a reflection of your abilities or worth as a person. They are simply part of the journey and should not define you or your progress. Remember that everyone makes mistakes and faces challenges, and it's okay to stumble along the way. The most important thing is to pick yourself back up, learn from your mistakes, and keep moving forward.

A positive mindset and a growth-oriented attitude can help you overcome setbacks and stay motivated on your journey to a healthy lifestyle. Surround yourself with supportive people who will encourage you and help you stay focused on your goals. And most importantly, be patient and kind to yourself. A healthy lifestyle is a journey, not a destination, and it takes time, effort, and dedication to achieve.

Here's a workbook exercise to help avoid and cope with setbacks

1. Introduction: Take a moment to reflect on your own experiences with setbacks in your journey to a healthy lifestyle. Write down any instances where you faced obstacles or challenges and how you responded to them.

2. Reframing Setbacks: In this exercise, you will reframe your perspective on setbacks. Reflect on the following statements:
-Setbacks are not a reflection of my abilities or worth.
-Setbacks are opportunities for growth and learning.
-I can learn from my mistakes and do things differently next time.

3. Analyzing Setbacks: For each setback you wrote down in the introduction, answer the following questions:

- What was the setback?
- How did it make you feel?
- What can you do differently next time to avoid similar setbacks?

4. Moving Forward: Write down your action plan for moving forward after a setback. Include steps you can take to stay motivated, overcome obstacles, and stay focused on your goals.

5. Final Reflection: Take a moment to reflect on what you learned from this exercise. Write down how you will apply these lessons to your journey to a healthy lifestyle moving forward.

Remember, setbacks are a normal part of the journey, and it's important to not let them discourage you. By reframing your perspective and learning from your mistakes, you can stay motivated and keep moving forward towards your goals.

Maintaining Your Mindset for Long-Term Weight Loss

Maintaining a positive mindset is key to achieving and sustaining long-term weight loss. Here are some practical tips for maintaining a healthy weight loss mindset:

1. Practice gratitude: Take time each day to focus on what you are grateful for, including your progress and accomplishments in your weight loss journey.
Stay positive: Surround yourself with positive people and situa-tions, and try to focus on the good in every situation.

2. Stay active: Regular physical activity can help boost your mood, reduce stress, and maintain a healthy weight.

3. Eat a balanced diet: Eating a balanced diet that includes a variety of healthy foods can help you feel satisfied and energized, and reduce the risk of emotional eating.

5. Get enough sleep: Adequate sleep is important for physical and mental health, and can help regulate hormones that affect hunger and metabolism.

6. Manage stress: Find healthy ways to manage stress, such as through exercise, meditation, or deep breathing.

7. Be patient: Weight loss is a gradual process, and it is important to be patient and celebrate small victories along the way.

8. Avoid comparing yourself to others: Everyone's weight loss journey is unique, and it is important to focus on your own progress and goals, rather than comparing yourself to others.

9. Stay accountable: Find a support system, such as a friend, family member, or weight loss support group, to help hold you account-able and provide encouragement.

By incorporating these tips into your daily routine, you can maintain a positive and healthy mindset throughout your weight loss journey. Remember, the journey to a healthier weight is not just about the numbers on the scale, but also about the positive changes you are making in your life and the person you are becoming.

Here's a simple workbook exercise to help you maintain a healthy weight loss mindset:

1. Reflection: Take a few moments to reflect on your weight loss journey so far. What have been some of your biggest challenges and successes? What do you feel are the most important factors for maintaining a positive weight loss mindset?

2. Gratitude: In the next page, make a list of things you are grateful for. This can include your progress in your weight loss journey, your support system, and your health. Try to add to this list each day.

3. Positive Thinking: On the next page, write down positive affirmations or quotes that inspire you. Read these affirmations every day to help maintain a positive mindset.

4. Physical Activity: On the next page, create a weekly exercise plan. Include the type of physical activity you will do, the duration, and the days of the week.

5. Healthy Eating: On the next page, create a meal plan for the week. Make sure to include a variety of healthy foods, and don't forget to treat yourself every once in a while!

6. Sleep: On the next page, write down your bedtime routine. Make sure to include relaxing activities, such as reading or listening to music, to help you wind down before bed.

7. Stress Management: On the next page, write down healthy ways to manage stress. This can include exercise, meditation, deep breathing, or spending time with loved ones.

8. Patience: On the next page, write down a reminder to be patient with yourself and your weight loss journey. Celebrate small victories along the way, and remember that weight loss is a gradual process.

9. Accountability: On the next page, write down the names of people in your support system. Reach out to them for encouragement and accountability when you need it.

10. Celebrations: On the final page, make a list of upcoming events or milestones to celebrate. This can include reaching a weight loss goal, fitting into a new outfit, or simply making healthy choices every day.

Recap of the Skinny Mindset Principles

The Skinny Mindset is a holistic approach to weight loss and healthy living. This approach challenges the traditional mindset of dieting and focuses on creating a positive and empowering relationship with food, exercise, and our bodies.

The Skinny Mindset is based on the following principles:

1. Mindset Shift: The first step in achieving a skinny mindset is to shift our focus from external factors such as diet and exercise to internal factors such as our thoughts and beliefs. This means recognizing and challenging negative self-talk and developing a positive relationship with our bodies and food.

2. Emotional Eating: Emotional eating is a common problem that can sabotage weight loss efforts. The Skinny Mindset teaches us torecognize and manage our emotions, rather than turning to food for comfort. This involves developing a deeper understanding of our emotions and finding alternative ways to cope with them.

3. Mindful Eating: Mindful eating is a key aspect of the Skinny Mindset. This involves being fully present and aware while eating, paying attention to hunger and fullness signals, and savoring each bite. By practicing mindful eating, we can break the cycle of emotional eating and develop a healthier relationship with food.

4. Eating for Nourishment: The Skinny Mindset encourages us to focus on nourishing our bodies with nutrient-dense foods, rather than restricting certain foods or counting calories. This approach helps us to establish a healthy relationship with food and avoid the yo-yo dieting cycle.

5. Exercise for Health: Exercise is an important aspect of the Skinny Mindset, but it is not the focus. Instead of using exercise as a means to burn calories or punish ourselves for eating, we are encouraged to view it as a way to improve our overall health and well-being.

6. Body Acceptance: The Skinny Mindset teaches us to accept and love our bodies, regardless of size or shape. This involves breaking free from societal beauty standards and embracing our unique bodies. By accepting and loving our bodies, we can break free from the cycle of dieting and develop a positive and empowering relationship with food and exercise.

7. Self-Care: Self-care is a crucial component of the Skinny Mindset. This involves taking care of our physical, emotional, and mental well-being. This includes activities such as getting enough sleep, practicing self-compassion, and engaging in activities that bring us joy.

Space for your thoughts:

Final Thoughts and Encouragement

Congratulations on reaching the end of "Skinny Mindset." I hope that throughout this book, you have learned valuable insights and tips to help you develop a healthy relationship with food, exercise, and your body.

It is important to remember that this journey is not easy and it is normal to encounter challenges along the way. However, we encourage you to be patient with yourself and to celebrate your progress, no matter how small it may be.

I also want to emphasize that your worth is not determined by your body size or shape. It is important to focus on developing a positive self-image and to practice self-compassion. This can include accepting and loving yourself just as you are, and being kind to yourself when you make mistakes or fall off track.

In conclusion, I want to remind you that skinny is not the only definition of beauty or health. It is essential to strive for a healthy lifestyle and mindset, but not at the expense of your well-being. The goal is to find balance and to live a life filled with joy, happiness, and self-acceptance.

I hope that "Skinny Mindset" has inspired and empowered you to take control of your thoughts and habits, and to achieve your health and wellness goals in a sustainable and fulfilling way. We wish you all the best on your journey and remember, be kind to yourself and always celebrate your progress.

Thank you and well done!

					Meal Time
					Location and company
					Type of food and drink
					Hunger on a scale from 0 to 10
					Feelings before eating
					Feelings after eating
					Reflections

					Meal Time
					Location and company
					Type of food and drink
					Hunger on a scale from 0 to 10
					Feelings before eating
					Feelings after eating
					Reflections

					Meal Time
					Location and company
					Type of food and drink
					Hunger on a scale from 0 to 10
					Feelings before eating
					Feelings after eating
					Reflections

Meal Time	Location and company	Type of food and drink	Hunger on a scale from 0 to 10	Feelings before eating	Feelings after eating	Reflections

					Meal Time
					Location and company
					Type of food and drink
					Hunger on a scale from 0 to 10
					Feelings before eating
					Feelings after eating
					Reflections

Meal Time	Location and company	Type of food and drink	Hunger on a scale from 0 to 10	Feelings before eating	Feelings after eating	Reflections

					Meal Time
					Location and company
					Type of food and drink
					Hunger on a scale from 0 to 10
					Feelings before eating
					Feelings after eating
					Reflections

Printed in Great Britain
by Amazon